The Pain-Free Core Solution

Kettlebell Windmills for a Strong, Stable Midsection

Helen Talbott

Table of contents

Disclaimer
About the author
Anatomy of the Windmill: Muscles Targeted and Movement Breakdown
The Perfect Setup: Form Cues and Common Mistakes to Avoid
The Perfect Setup: Form Cues and Common Mistakes to Avoid
Windmilling with Ease: Step-by-Step Guide with Variations
Building Consistency: Programming and Sample Workouts for All Levels
Identifying and Addressing Common Core Pain Sources
Mobility and Flexibility Drills for Optimal Windmill Performance
Core Activation Techniques: Engaging Your Deep Core Muscles
Breathing and Bracing for Stability: Optimizing Your Core Connection
Recovery and Maintenance: Essential Practices for Long-Term Windmill Success

Synergistic Exercises: Complementing the Windmill with Other Core Workouts
Functional Core Training: Integrating Windmills into Daily Activities and Sports
Advanced Windmill Variations: Pushing Your Limits Safely and Effectively
Staying Motivated: Tips and Strategies for Long-Term Adherence
Conclusion: Building a Strong, Stable, and Pain-Free Core with Kettlebell Windmills
Request for a review

Disclaimer

This book is intended for informational purposes only and should not be construed as medical advice.

The information contained within this book should not be used to diagnose, treat, or prevent any medical condition. Please consult with a qualified healthcare professional before starting any new exercise program, especially if you have any pre-existing injuries or medical conditions.

Exercise and fitness activities can be inherently dangerous and carry the risk of injury. The author and publisher of this book disclaim any liability or responsibility for any injuries or damages that may arise from the use of the information contained herein.

It is important to listen to your body and stop any exercise that causes pain or discomfort. If you experience any pain or discomfort, please consult with a healthcare professional immediately.

The results of the exercises and techniques described in this book may vary from person to person. Individual factors such as age, fitness level, and previous injuries can all affect the results.

This book is not a substitute for professional guidance. It is recommended that you consult with a certified personal trainer or qualified healthcare professional to create a personalized exercise program that is tailored to your individual needs and goals.

Always use proper form and technique when performing the exercises described in this book. Incorrect form can increase your risk of injury. If you are unsure about the proper form, please consult with a qualified professional.

The use of kettlebells has inherent risks and requires proper instruction and safety precautions. Please ensure you understand the risks and proper techniques before using kettlebells.

By using this book, you agree to and accept the terms of this disclaimer.

Additional Recommendations:

- Consult with a healthcare professional before starting any new exercise program, especially if you have any pre-existing injuries or medical conditions.
- Be aware of your limitations and start slowly, gradually increasing the intensity and duration of your workouts as you get stronger.
- Always use proper form and technique to avoid injury.
- Listen to your body and stop any exercise that causes pain or discomfort.

- Seek professional guidance if you are unsure about anything.

About the author

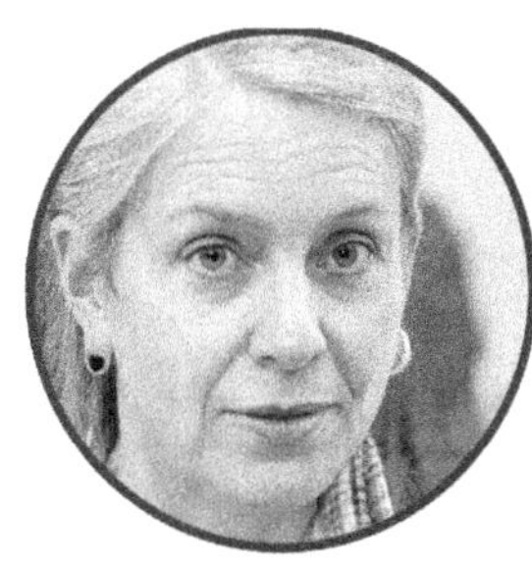

Helen Talbott is a passionate advocate for core health and a firm believer in the transformative power of the Kettlebell Windmill. As a certified personal trainer, she has witnessed firsthand the incredible results this exercise can achieve, helping countless individuals overcome pain, build strength, and unlock a newfound freedom of movement.

Driven by a desire to empower others and share her knowledge, Helen embarked on a mission to create The Pain-Free Core Solution: Kettlebell Windmills for a Strong, Stable Midsection. Drawing on her extensive experience and expertise, she meticulously crafted this comprehensive guide to equip readers with everything they need to conquer the Windmill and unlock the secrets to a strong, stable, and pain-free core.

Beyond her qualifications and experience, Helen is:

- A lifelong athlete: Her passion for movement and fitness stems from years of personal experience in various sports and disciplines.
- A dedicated researcher: She continuously stays updated on the latest research and advancements in fitness and core training, ensuring her approach is evidence-based and effective.
- An empathetic coach: Helen understands the challenges and obstacles people face on their fitness journeys. Her writing style is approachable, encouraging, and full of practical advice.
- A motivational force: Helen's enthusiasm and genuine desire to help others shine through her writing, inspiring readers to embrace the Windmill and achieve their core strength goals.

When you pick up "The Pain-Free Core Solution," you're not just getting a book; you're gaining a knowledgeable guide, a supportive coach, and a partner on your journey to a stronger, pain-free you.

Introduction

Escape the Pain Cycle, Unleash Your Core
Potential

Have you ever reached for that "dream bod" only to be met with a nagging pain in your lower back, hips, or glutes? Or maybe you're tired of endless crunches that deliver minimal results. If so, you're not alone. Countless individuals struggle with painful core issues that limit their fitness journey and overall well-being.

But what if there was a solution that not only sculpted a strong, stable core but also addressed the root cause of your pain?

Enter the Kettlebell Windmill: a transformative exercise that transcends the limitations of traditional core training. This powerful movement, often dubbed the "anti-crunch," combines strength, flexibility, and mobility to unlock a deep, functional core that's both resilient and pain-free.

This book is your guide to unlocking the transformative power of the Kettlebell Windmill. Whether you're a fitness newcomer or a seasoned athlete battling chronic pain, this comprehensive guide will empower you to:

- Ditch the pain: Learn the science behind pain-free core training and identify the root causes of your discomfort.
- Master the Windmill: Demystify the movement with detailed breakdowns, form cues, and progressions tailored to your needs.
- Build a strong, stable core: Discover how the Windmill engages your entire

core for unmatched strength, stability, and functional performance.

- Move with freedom: Improve mobility and flexibility for effortless Windmills and pain-free everyday movement.
- Go beyond the basics: Explore advanced variations, synergistic exercises, and programing strategies to keep your core challenged and engaged.
- Stay motivated: Learn practical tips and strategies to stay committed to your core journey and achieve lasting results.

This is not just another workout book. It's a roadmap to reclaiming your core and unleashing a pain-free, stronger, and more confident you. Are you ready to embark on this transformative journey? Turn the page and begin your Windmill adventure!

Why the Kettlebell Windmill? Unveiling the Core-Strengthening Powerhouse

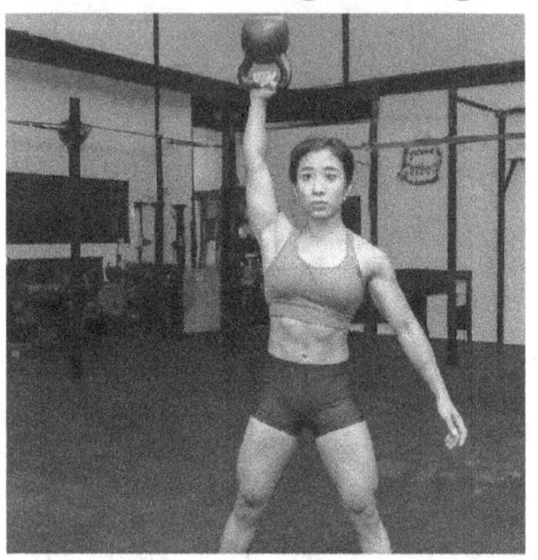

For years, crunches and planks have reigned supreme in the domain of core training. But what if there was a more efficient, versatile, and even pain-free way to unlock a truly strong and stable core? Enter the Kettlebell Windmill, a movement poised to revolutionize your core workouts and redefine what it means to have a healthy midsection.

Ditch the Monotony, Embrace Versatility:

Unlike crunches that isolate specific muscles, the Windmill is a multi-planar movement, engaging your entire core through a dynamic hip hinge, rotation, and overhead press. This holistic approach simultaneously strengthens your abs, obliques, glutes, hamstrings, shoulders, and back, creating a foundation of functional strength that translates to everyday life and athletic performance.

Strength Beyond Definition:

Forget the chiseled six-pack ideal. The Windmill prioritizes deep core activation, targeting the muscles responsible for spinal stability and proper movement mechanics. This translates to a core that's not just aesthetically pleasing, but also resilient and injury-resistant. No more aching lower back from lifting groceries or worrying about pain during your favorite sport.

Pain-Free Core: A Radical Shift:

Traditional core exercises often exacerbate existing pain due to their isolation focus and unnatural positions. The Windmill, however, adopts a pain-friendly approach, prioritizing proper form and alignment. Additionally, its focus on mobility and flexibility helps address tightness and imbalances that contribute to pain in the first place.

Embrace the Challenge, Reap the Rewards:

Mastering the Windmill requires dedication and practice, but the journey itself is rewarding. This dynamic movement keeps your mind and body engaged, while the feeling of a strong, stable core motivates you to push further. Soon, you'll not only see physical results but also experience improved balance, posture, and confidence in your movements.

Are you ready to ditch the pain, unlock your core potential, and experience the transformative power of the Kettlebell Windmill? Turn the page and embark on your journey to a stronger, healthier, and pain-free you!

Understanding Pain-Free Core Training: Principles and Benefits

For decades, "core training" has conjured images of endless crunches and plank variations, often leaving us with sore backs and little progress. The good news? There's a better way. Pain-free core training focuses on building a strong, stable, and functional core without the discomfort or risk of injury associated with traditional methods.

Core Misconceptions Debunked:

- Myth: Strong abs = six-pack definition.
- Truth: Deep core muscles, responsible for stability and proper movement, often lie beneath the six-pack and are crucial for pain-free movement.
- Myth: Crunches are king.

- Truth: Crunches isolate specific muscles, neglecting the holistic core system and potentially causing imbalances.
- Myth: No pain, no gain.
- Truth: Pain during core exercises often indicates improper form or underlying issues. Pain-free training prioritizes alignment and movement quality for safe and sustainable results.

Principles of Pain-Free Core Training:

- Functional movement: Exercises mimicking real-life activities, like the Windmill, engage multiple muscle groups and promote transferable strength.
- Mind-muscle connection: Focusing on activating deep core muscles rather than relying solely on external

movement ensures optimal engagement.

- Mobility and flexibility: Addressing tight muscles and joint limitations creates a foundation for proper core activation and pain-free movement.
- Gradual progression: Starting with bodyweight exercises and progressions helps prevent strain and allows for safe advancement.
- Proper form and alignment: Avoiding excessive spinal flexion and maintaining neutral spine position minimizes stress on the back.
- Breathing and bracing: Integrating proper breathing techniques with core engagement enhances stability and core activation.

Benefits of Pain-Free Core Training:

- Reduced pain: Addresses imbalances and weaknesses that contribute to back pain and discomfort.
- Improved posture and alignment: Strong core stabilizes the spine, leading to better posture and reduced risk of injury.
- Enhanced athletic performance: Increased core strength translates to better power, balance, and coordination in sports and activities.
- Functional movement efficiency: Improved core stability translates to smoother, more efficient movements in daily life.
- Boosted confidence: Feeling strong and stable in your core can improve overall confidence and well-being.

Ready to embrace pain-free core training and unlock its benefits? This book will equip you with the knowledge, exercises, and strategies

to build a strong, stable, and pain-free core
for life!

Who is this Book For? Addressing Different Fitness Levels and Pain Concerns

Whether you're a seasoned athlete or a complete fitness newbie, struggling with chronic pain or pain-free and eager to explore, this book is for YOU if you want to build a strong, stable, and pain-free core using the transformative power of the Kettlebell Windmill.

If you identify with any of the following, this book will be your valuable guide:

New to Exercise:

- You're eager to begin your fitness journey and prioritize a strong core.

- You're intimidated by complex gym routines and prefer functional, bodyweight-based exercises.

- You're looking for a safe and effective way to build core strength without risking injury.

Fitness Enthusiasts:

- You're looking for a fresh challenge to elevate your core workouts beyond crunches and planks.

- You want to improve functional strength and stability for better performance in your chosen sport or activity.

- You're interested in diversifying your workout routine and exploring new movement patterns.

Dealing with Pain:

- You experience chronic pain in your lower back, hips, or glutes that limits your core exercises.

- You're concerned about traditional core exercises exacerbating your pain and want pain-free alternatives.

- You're looking for a holistic approach to core training that addresses the root cause of your pain.

Regardless of your current fitness level or pain concerns, this book:

- Offers clear modifications and progressions to tailor the Windmill to your individual needs and abilities.

- Provides pain-free core training principles and strategies to ensure safe and effective exercise.

- Addresses common concerns and offers modifications for various pain conditions.

- Empowers you to build a strong, stable, and functional core that supports your overall well-being.

Remember, the journey to a stronger, pain-free core is yours to own. This book equips you with the knowledge and tools to embark on that journey, embrace the transformative power of the Windmill, and achieve your fitness goals!

Chapter 1

Anatomy of the Windmill: Muscles Targeted and Movement Breakdown

Welcome to the heart of the Kettlebell Windmill! In this chapter, we'll embark on a journey of understanding the movement's intricacies, dissecting the muscles it engages, and analyzing its various phases. This knowledge will empower you to perform the Windmill with confidence, maximizing its benefits and minimizing any risk of injury.

Muscles in Action:

Imagine the Windmill as a symphony of muscles working in harmony. While the entire body participates, some key players deserve our focus:

- Core: The unsung hero! Rectus abdominis, obliques, transverse abdominis, and the elusive pelvic floor all join forces to provide spinal stability, rotational power, and anti-extension support throughout the movement.

- Posterior Chain: Glutes, hamstrings, and erector spinae form the powerhouse, responsible for hip hinging, knee extension, and maintaining a neutral spine.

- Shoulders & Upper Back: Rotator cuff muscles, rhomboids, and lats stabilize the shoulder joint and contribute to overhead pressing and reaching.

Deconstructing the Movement:

The Windmill can be broken down into distinct phases, each targeting specific muscle groups:

1. The Setup:

- Standing tall with a neutral spine, engage your core and prepare to receive the kettlebell.
- Hinge at the hips, maintaining a flat back and pushing your hips back as if to sit in a chair.

- Grasp the kettlebell with one hand, arm extended overhead. This activates your lats and shoulder stabilizers.

2. **The Descent**:

- Continue hinging deeper, allowing the torso to rotate towards the opposite leg. Your free hand reaches towards the ground for balance, engaging obliques and core stabilizers.

- Feel the stretch in your hamstrings and glutes as you reach your deepest point.

3. **The Ascend**:

- Engage your core and glutes to initiate the upward movement.

- Press the kettlebell overhead, activating your shoulders and triceps.
- Rotate your torso back to upright, feeling the obliques and core work to stabilize.

- Return to the starting position, maintaining a strong, neutral spine.

Remember: This is a simplified breakdown. Each phase involves intricate interplay between various muscles. With practice and focused attention, you'll cultivate a deeper understanding of your body's mechanics during the Windmill.

Next Steps:

In the next chapter, we'll delve into choosing the right kettlebell weight and explore safe progressions.

Stay tuned for detailed form cues and common mistakes to avoid, ensuring you master the Windmill with precision and grace.

Are you ready to unlock the true potential of the Windmill? Turn the page and let's begin your core transformation!

Chapter 2
Choosing the Right Kettlebell: Weight Selection and Progressions

Now that you've unlocked the anatomical secrets of the Windmill, it's time to choose your weapon: the kettlebell. But wait, with numerous weights staring back at you, how do you select the perfect one? Worry not, for this chapter guides you through weight selection and safe progressions, ensuring your Windmill journey starts on the right foot (or should we say, hip hinge?).

Finding Your Starting Point:

Forget about ego lifting! When it comes to the Windmill, prioritizing form and control over heavy weights is key. Here's how to choose your starting kettlebell:

- Beginners: Opt for a light kettlebell. Lighter weights (5-10lbs) allow you to focus on form, build core strength, and minimize injury risk.

- Intermediate: If you have some fitness experience, a moderate kettlebell (12-15lbs) might be suitable.

- Advanced: Experienced lifters can choose a heavier kettlebell (18-25lbs or more). However, prioritize form over max weight and adjust as needed.

Remember: These are just general guidelines. It's always best to start lighter and gradually increase weight as you master the movement. Listen to your body and prioritize perfect form over heavier weights.

Progression Pathways:

As you conquer the Windmill with a specific weight, it's time to challenge yourself further. Here are safe and effective ways to progress:

- Increase Weight: Once you can perform the Windmill with perfect form for several sets, consider gradually increasing the kettlebell weight by 2-5lbs.

- Hold for Longer: Extend the hold at the bottom of the movement, challenging your core stability and isometric strength.

- Change Hand Positions: Once comfortable with single-handed variations, try the "two-handed windmill" for a different core engagement.

- Introduce Variations: Explore advanced variations like the "traveling windmill" or the "pistol windmill" for an extra challenge (ensure proper guidance first).

Always remember: Progress gradually, pay attention to your body's signals, and prioritize proper form above all else. If you experience pain or discomfort, reduce the weight, modify the exercise, or seek professional guidance.

Next Steps:

In the next chapter, we'll delve into the nitty-gritty of the Windmill with detailed form cues and common mistakes to avoid.
Stay tuned for strategies to conquer the Windmill with precision and elegance, paving the way for a strong, stable, and pain-free core!

Ready to embark on your weight-selection journey and unlock the next level of your Windmill? Turn the page and let's conquer the kettlebell together!

Chapter 3

The Perfect Setup: Form Cues and Common Mistakes to Avoid

Mastering the Windmill requires more than just throwing a kettlebell around. It's a dance of precision, where every detail matters. In this chapter, we'll equip you with the essential form cues and highlight common mistakes to avoid, ensuring your Windmill journey is safe, effective, and pain-free.

Setting the Stage for Success:

- Foot Position: Plant your feet hip-width apart, toes slightly angled away from the kettlebell side. This creates a stable base for the movement.

- Posture Check: Maintain a tall spine with a neutral arch in your lower back. Avoid rounding your shoulders or collapsing inwards.
- Core Engagement: Brace your core as if preparing for a punch. Imagine pulling your belly button towards your spine for optimal stability.

- Kettlebell Grip: Grasp the kettlebell firmly with one hand, arm extended overhead. Ensure a neutral wrist position and avoid excessive gripping.

The Descent Symphony:

- Hinge, Don't Squat: Initiate the movement by hinging at your hips, pushing your hips back as if sitting in a chair. Avoid bending your knees excessively.

- Rotate with Control: As you hinge, allow your torso to rotate naturally towards the opposite leg. Don't force the rotation, but listen to your body's movement.

- Eyes on the Prize: Keep your gaze focused on a point in front of you, maintaining a neutral head and neck position. Avoid looking down at the floor.

- Free Hand Assist: Use your free hand for balance and guidance, reaching towards the ground without placing full weight on it.

The Ascend and Return:

- Press with Power: Engage your legs, glutes, and core to press the kettlebell overhead, maintaining a straight arm and engaged shoulder.

- Reverse the Rotation: As you ascend, rotate your torso back to upright, feeling your core muscles work to stabilize your spine.

- Finish Strong: Return to the starting position with a controlled movement, maintaining proper posture and core engagement throughout.

Mistakes to Leave Behind:

- Hunching Back: Avoid rounding your shoulders or collapsing your spine at any point during the movement.

- Knee Bending Frenzy: Remember, hinging prioritizes hip movement, not excessive knee bending.

- Looking for Your Shoes: Keep your gaze forward to maintain balance and avoid neck strain.

- Ego Lifting: Start light and prioritize form over heavy weights. Injury is not a badge of honor in the Windmill world.

- Forgetting to Breathe: Breathe naturally throughout the movement. Don't hold your breath or strain your neck.

Remember: Mastering form takes time and practice. Be patient, focus on the cues, and don't hesitate to seek professional guidance if needed.

Next Steps:

- In the next chapter, we'll delve into step-by-step instructions for the Windmill, accompanied by helpful imagery to solidify your understanding.

- Stay tuned for a variety of Windmill variations and programming strategies to keep your core challenged and engaged!

Ready to refine your Windmill technique and avoid common pitfalls? Turn the page and let's build a strong, stable, and pain-free core together!

Chapter 4

Windmilling with Ease: Step-by-Step Guide with Variations

Now that you've grasped the anatomy, chosen your weight, and honed your form, it's time to unveil the magic! This chapter provides a detailed, step-by-step guide for the Windmill, equipping you with the confidence and knowledge to execute the movement with grace and power. We'll also explore exciting variations to keep your core challenged and engaged.

Step-by-Step Windmill Mastery:

1. Prepare for Launch: Choose your kettlebell, stand tall with proper foot

positioning, engage your core, and extend one arm overhead holding the kettlebell.

2. Initiate the Hinge: Push your hips back as if sitting in a chair, maintaining a neutral spine and avoiding excessive knee bend.

3. Rotate and Reach: As you hinge, allow your torso to naturally rotate towards the opposite leg. Extend your free hand towards the ground for balance, keeping your gaze forward.

4. Descent with Control: Continue hinging deeper until you reach your comfortable maximum depth, feeling a stretch in your hamstrings and glutes. Maintain a tall spine and core engagement throughout.

5. Ascend with Power: Engage your core and glutes to press the kettlebell overhead, ensuring a straight arm and stable shoulder.

6. Reverse the Rotation: As you ascend, rotate your torso back to upright, feeling your obliques and core work to stabilize your spine.

7. Return to Base: Lower the kettlebell to the starting position with control, maintaining proper posture and core engagement.

8. Repeat on Both Sides: Complete the same steps on the other side, challenging your body with balanced core development.

Pro Tips:

- Visualize the movement as a coordinated hinge, rotation, and press, rather than isolated actions.

- Breathe naturally throughout the movement, avoiding holding your breath.

- Start slow and gradually increase your pace as you become comfortable with the form.

- Don't forget to warm up before your Windmill workout and cool down afterward.

Variations to Spice Up Your Routine:

- Two-Handed Windmill: Hold the kettlebell with both hands overhead for a different core engagement.

- Traveling Windmill: Take a small step to the side as you perform the Windmill, adding an element of balance and coordination.

- Pistol Windmill: Perform the Windmill while balancing on one leg for a unilateral core challenge (advanced!).

- Offset Windmill: Hold the kettlebell offset from your body for an additional rotational challenge.

Remember: Choose variations that suit your fitness level and always prioritize proper form over complexity.

Next Steps:

- In the next chapter, we'll dive into the world of pain-free core training, addressing common concerns and offering strategies for a holistic approach.

- Stay tuned for sample workouts and programming tips to integrate the Windmill into your fitness routine seamlessly!

Ready to set your core ablaze with the Windmill and its exciting variations? Turn the page and embark on a journey of strength, stability, and pain-free movement!

Chapter 5

Building Consistency: Programming and Sample Workouts for All Levels

Conquering the Windmill is just the beginning. To truly unlock its transformative potential, consistent practice is key. This chapter delves into the world of programming and sample workouts, empowering you to create a personalized plan that fits your fitness level and goals. Remember, consistency is the magic ingredient for building a strong, stable, and pain-free core!

Crafting Your Core Blueprint:

- Frequency: Aim for 2-3 Windmill workouts per week, allowing adequate rest for muscle recovery.
- Sets and Reps: Beginners can start with 2-3 sets of 5-8 repetitions per side. Gradually increase as you gain strength and confidence.
- Intensity: Choose a kettlebell weight that challenges you without compromising form. Focus on quality repetitions over heavy weights.
- Progression: Incorporate variations, increase weight, or try longer holds at the bottom of the movement to keep your core challenged.
- Warm-up and Cool-down: Don't neglect these crucial steps to prevent injury and optimize performance.

Sample Workouts for Different Levels:

Beginner:

- Warm-up: 5 minutes of light cardio and dynamic stretches
- Windmill: 2 sets of 5-8 repetitions per side with a light kettlebell
- Core Plank: 3 sets of 30-60 seconds hold
- Cool-down: Static stretches and deep breathing

Intermediate:

- Warm-up: 10 minutes of dynamic stretches and mobility drills
- Windmill: 3 sets of 8-12 repetitions per side with a moderate kettlebell
- Anti-Rotational Press: 3 sets of 10 repetitions per side
- Bird Dog: 3 sets of 10 repetitions per side
- Cool-down: Static stretches and foam rolling

Advanced:

- Warm-up: 15 minutes of dynamic stretches and light cardio with mobility drills
- Traveling Windmill: 3 sets of 6-8 repetitions per side with a challenging kettlebell
- Pistol Windmill: 2 sets of 5 repetitions per side (alternate legs)
- Hanging Leg Raise: 3 sets of max repetitions
- Cool-down: Static stretches and self-massage

Remember: These are just examples. Adapt the workouts based on your needs and preferences. Consult a fitness professional for personalized guidance.

Beyond the Windmill:

Remember, the Windmill is a powerful tool within a holistic core training approach. Consider incorporating other exercises that target different core muscles and movement patterns for a well-rounded core workout:

- Planks and variations
- Deadbugs and hollow holds
- Anti-rotational exercises
- Loaded carries and farmers walks

Embrace the Journey:

Building a strong, stable, and pain-free core takes time and dedication. Celebrate your progress, listen to your body, and most importantly, enjoy the journey! With consistent practice and the Windmill as your guide, you're well on your way to achieving your core fitness goals.

Now go forth and conquer your core!

Chapter 6

Identifying and Addressing Common Core Pain Sources

While the Windmill promises a strong, stable, and pain-free core, pre-existing pain can cast a shadow. This chapter delves into common core pain sources, guiding you in identifying the culprit and offering strategies to address it, paving the way for pain-free Windmill training.

Unveiling the Painful Culprits:

- Lower Back Pain: Often stemming from imbalances, weak core muscles, or improper form in exercises.

- Hip Pain: Tightness in hip flexors or gluteal imbalances can contribute to hip pain during core work.
- Sciatica: This radiating pain down the leg can sometimes be triggered by core exercises due to nerve impingement.
- Groin Pain: Inflammation in the adductor muscles, often caused by overexertion or improper exercise technique.
- Pelvic Floor Dysfunction: Weakened or overly tight pelvic floor muscles can contribute to various pain and discomfort in the core region.

Remember: This list is not exhaustive, and seeking professional medical advice is crucial for accurate diagnosis and treatment of pain.

Finding Your Pain Point:

- Location: Pinpoint the exact location and nature of the pain (sharp, dull, aching).
- Onset: Identify when the pain occurs (during specific exercises, throughout the day).
- Aggravating factors: Analyze movements or activities that worsen the pain.
- Medical history: Consider any pre-existing conditions or injuries that might contribute.

Combating the Pain:

- Rest and Recovery: Allow your body time to heal, especially when experiencing acute pain.
- Movement Modification: Explore pain-free variations of core exercises, like bodyweight Windmills or plank modifications.
- Stretching and Mobility: Address tight muscles and improve flexibility, especially hip flexors, hamstrings, and glutes.
- Strengthening: Once pain-free, gradually introduce core strengthening exercises that target weaker muscle groups.
- Proper form: Seek professional guidance to ensure proper form and

technique in all exercises, including the Windmill.

- Myofascial release: Self-massage with foam rollers or balls can help release trigger points and muscle tension.
- Consider alternative therapies: Depending on the pain source, physical therapy, yoga, or Pilates can offer targeted solutions.

Remember: Listen to your body and prioritize pain-free movement. Don't push through pain, and adapt your workouts to accommodate your healing process.

Next Steps:

In the next chapter, we'll explore mobility and flexibility drills specifically designed to support pain-free Windmill execution.

- Stay tuned for core activation techniques and breathing strategies to optimize your core engagement and minimize pain risk.

- Ready to identify and address the root cause of your core pain, paving the way for a joyful Windmill journey? Turn the page and unlock the door to pain-free movement!

Chapter 7

Mobility and Flexibility Drills for Optimal Windmill Performance

Unleashing the true power of the Windmill demands not just strength, but also mobility and flexibility. Tight muscles and limited range of motion can hinder your form, increase your risk of injury, and prevent you from reaping the full benefits of this transformative exercise. This chapter equips you with essential mobility and flexibility drills, paving the way for a pain-free, graceful, and powerful Windmill.

Mobility Essentials:

- Hip flexor stretch: Kneel on one leg, lunge the other leg forward, and gently push your hips forward until you feel a stretch in your front thigh. Hold for 30 seconds and repeat on the other side.

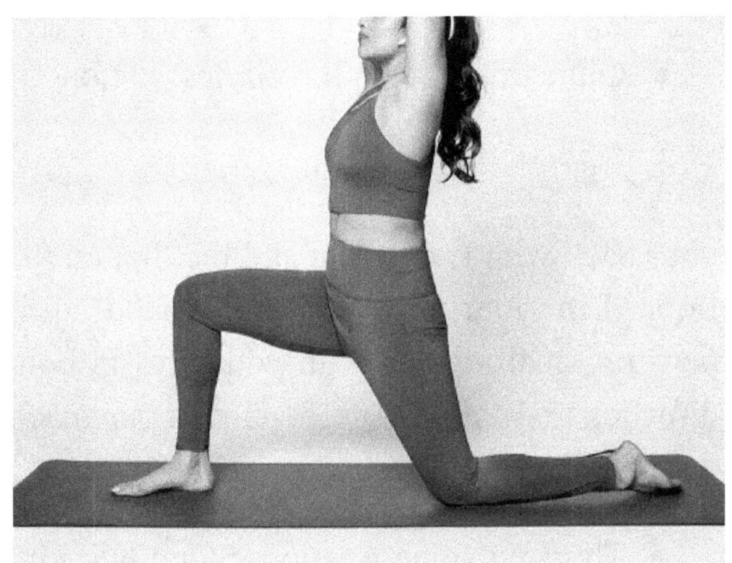

- Glute bridge with hip circles: Lie on

your back with knees bent and feet flat on the floor. Lift your hips off the ground, then perform small circles with your hips in both directions. Repeat 10-15 circles in each direction.

- Thoracic spine rotation: Stand tall with feet shoulder-width apart. Place your hands behind your back and gently rotate your upper body from side to side, feeling a stretch in your chest and spine. Hold for 5 seconds each side and repeat 5-10 times.

Flexibility Focus:

- Hamstring stretch: Sit on the floor with legs extended in front of you. Reach for your toes or as far down your legs as you can comfortably go, keeping your back straight. Hold for 30 seconds and repeat.

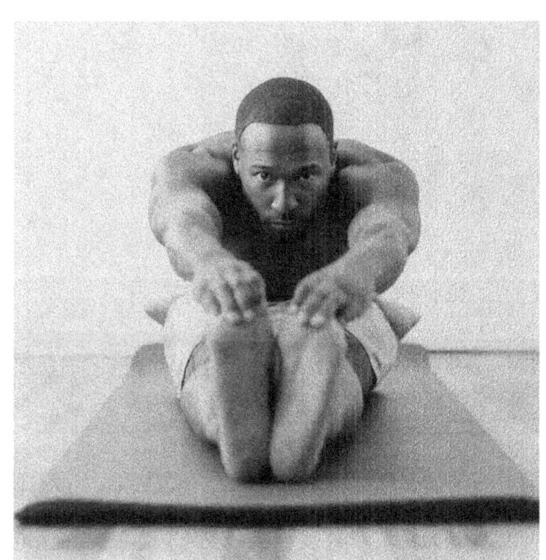

- Quadriceps stretch: Stand on one leg and hold onto a stable object for balance. Bend your other leg behind you and grab your foot or ankle, pulling your heel towards your buttocks. Hold for 30 seconds and repeat on the other side.

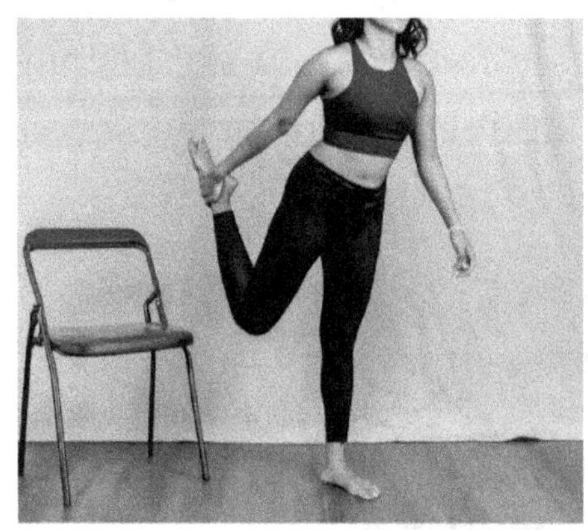

- Chest opener: Stand tall with arms overhead and fingers intertwined. Gently press your palms together, feeling a stretch in your chest and shoulders. Hold for 30 seconds and repeat.

Windmill-Specific Drills:

- Windmill arm circles: Hold a light kettlebell overhead and perform small circles with your arm in both directions. This mobilizes your shoulder joint and prepares it for the full Windmill movement.
- Windmill hinge practice: Focus on hinging at your hips while maintaining a long spine and neutral back. Practice this movement without the kettlebell first to ensure proper form.
- Windmill rotation drills: Stand with your feet hip-width apart and practice rotating your torso from side to side, mimicking the rotation in the Windmill. Gradually increase the range of motion as you feel comfortable.

Remember:

- Consistency is key! Aim for 5-10 minutes of mobility and flexibility drills several times a week, especially before your Windmill workouts.

- Listen to your body. Don't force any stretches or movements that cause pain.
- Focus on quality over quantity. Hold each stretch and drill for a sustained period to maximize its benefits.
- As your flexibility improves, you can gradually incorporate more challenging drills and variations.

Next Steps:

- In the next chapter, we'll delve into core activation techniques, ensuring your core muscles are primed and firing optimally during the Windmill.
- Stay tuned for breathing strategies and bracing techniques to enhance your core stability and performance.

Ready to unlock the full potential of your Windmill with the power of mobility and flexibility? Turn the page and embark on a journey of enhanced movement and pain-free core training!

Chapter 8

Core Activation Techniques: Engaging Your Deep Core Muscles

The Windmill demands not just strength, but also the coordinated activation of your deep core muscles. These hidden powerhouses, often neglected in traditional exercises, play a crucial role in stabilizing your spine, transferring force, and preventing injury. In this chapter, we unveil essential core activation techniques, ensuring your Windmill journey is fueled by a truly engaged and empowered core.

Unveiling the Deep Core:

Your deep core muscles, including the transverse abdominis, pelvic floor, and diaphragm, work together like an internal corset, providing stability and support from within. Activating them before and during the Windmill optimizes performance and minimizes the risk of pain.

Key Activation Techniques:

- Diaphragmatic Breathing: Engage your diaphragm, the dome-shaped muscle beneath your lungs, by inhaling deeply through your nose and feeling your belly expand. This creates intra-abdominal pressure, a crucial element for core stability.
- Pelvic Floor Activation: Imagine "lifting" your pelvic floor muscles as if stopping urine flow. Hold for a few seconds, then relax. Repeat this several times to enhance pelvic floor awareness and activation.
- Drawing In: Gently pull your belly button towards your spine without sucking in your stomach. This activates the transverse abdominis, a deep core muscle that provides spinal stability.
- Hollow Body Hold: Lie on your back with your lower back pressed into the ground,

lift your legs and shoulders slightly off the ground, and engage your core to maintain a "scooped" spine position. Hold for 30 seconds or as long as you can comfortably maintain the form.

Windmill Integration:

- Pre-Windmill Activation: Before initiating the Windmill, perform a few diaphragmatic breaths, pelvic floor squeezes, and drawing-in maneuvers. This primes your core muscles for optimal engagement.
- Maintain Activation Throughout: Throughout the Windmill, remember to keep your core engaged. Imagine drawing your belly button inward, maintaining a neutral spine, and using your diaphragm for breathing.
- Focus on Quality, Not Intensity: Don't clench your core excessively. Focus on feeling a light, sustained engagement as you move through the Windmill.

Remember:

- Core activation takes practice and consistency. Don't get discouraged if it doesn't feel natural at first. Keep practicing, and you'll gradually develop a strong mind-muscle connection with your deep core.
- If you experience any pain or discomfort, stop the exercise and consult a healthcare professional.

Next Steps:

- In the next chapter, we'll explore breathing strategies specifically designed to enhance core activation and optimize your Windmill performance.
- Stay tuned for bracing techniques that further stabilize your spine and core during the Windmill, empowering you to move with confidence and control.

Ready to unlock the hidden power of your deep core and elevate your Windmill experience? Turn the page and embark on a journey of core connection, stability, and pain-free movement!

Chapter 9

Breathing and Bracing for Stability: Optimizing Your Core Connection

We've explored core activation techniques, but for truly unlocking the Windmill's potential, you need to master the art of breathing and bracing. These seemingly simple actions become powerful tools when combined, creating a rock-solid core foundation for stability, power transfer, and injury prevention.

The Magic of Breathing:

Forget holding your breath during exercise! Diaphragmatic breathing, where you inhale deeply through your nose and exhale slowly through your mouth, engages your diaphragm, creates intra-abdominal pressure (IAP), and supports your spine from within.

Windmill Breathing Integration:

- Inhale as you hinge: As you initiate the Windmill's downward movement, take a deep diaphragmatic breath, feeling your belly expand.
- Exhale with control: As you ascend and press the kettlebell overhead, exhale slowly and steadily, maintaining IAP throughout the movement.
- Avoid breath holding: Holding your breath can strain your core and compromise stability. Breathe naturally and rhythmically throughout the Windmill.

The Power of Bracing:

Think of bracing as creating an internal "corset" with your core muscles. Imagine tightening your core as if preparing for a punch, engaging all layers of your abs, pelvic floor, and obliques.

Bracing for Windmill Success:

- Pre-bracing is key: Before initiating the Windmill, engage your core by bracing as if expecting a punch. Maintain this brace throughout the entire movement.
- Coordinate with breathing: Bracing works synergistically with breathing. Inhale as you brace, and exhale slowly while maintaining the brace.
- Focus on quality, not intensity: Don't clench your core excessively. Aim for a light, sustained brace that creates stability without compromising movement.

Remember:

- Breathing and bracing take practice and coordination. Don't get discouraged if it feels awkward at first. Keep practicing, and you'll develop a seamless integration of these techniques into your Windmill.

- Listen to your body. If you experience any discomfort, adjust your breathing or bracing, or rest if needed.

Next Steps:

- This concludes our exploration of the Windmill, its secrets, and its potential to transform your core. Remember, consistency is key! Keep practicing, stay motivated, and enjoy the journey towards a strong, stable, and pain-free core.
- As you progress, consider seeking personalized guidance from a qualified fitness professional to tailor your Windmill workouts and ensure optimal form and technique.

Ready to breathe, brace, and conquer the Windmill? You've got this! Remember, this is just the beginning of your core transformation journey. Embrace the challenge, celebrate your progress, and enjoy the power of movement!

Chapter 10

Recovery and Maintenance: Essential Practices for Long-Term Windmill Success

Conquering the Windmill is a thrilling feat, but like any physical endeavor, sustainable progress requires attention to recovery and maintenance. This chapter equips you with essential practices to ensure your body thrives on your Windmill journey, empowering you to reap the long-term benefits of a strong, stable, and pain-free core.

The Pillars of Recovery:

- Prioritize Rest: Listen to your body and schedule adequate rest days between Windmill workouts. Allow your muscles time to repair and rebuild, preventing overtraining and potential injuries.

- Embrace Sleep: Aim for 7-8 hours of quality sleep each night. Sleep is crucial for muscle recovery, hormonal balance, and cognitive function, all of which contribute to optimal Windmill performance and overall well-being.
- Fuel Your Body: Nourish your body with a balanced diet rich in fruits, vegetables, whole grains, and lean protein. Don't forget to stay hydrated by drinking plenty of water throughout the day. Proper nutrition provides the building blocks for muscle repair and fuels your training sessions.
- Active Recovery: Don't equate rest with stagnation. Engage in light activities like walking, yoga, or swimming on rest days to promote blood flow, aid recovery, and maintain mobility.
- Self-Massage: Invest in a foam roller or massage ball to release muscle tension, improve circulation, and reduce soreness. Consider self-massage before and after

workouts, focusing on areas particularly targeted by the Windmill.

Maintenance Matters:

- Warm-up and Cool-down: Never skip these crucial steps! Dynamic stretches and light cardio before your workouts prepare your body for movement, while static stretches and foam rolling afterwards promote cooldown and flexibility.
- Listen to Your Body: Pain is a signal, not a badge of honor. If you experience pain during the Windmill, adjust your form, reduce the weight, or rest until the pain subsides. Don't push through pain, as it can lead to injuries.
- Seek Professional Guidance: As you progress, consider consulting a certified personal trainer or physical therapist for personalized program design, form correction, and injury prevention strategies.

- Embrace Variety: While the Windmill remains your core focus, incorporate other core exercises and activities into your routine to challenge different muscle groups and prevent plateaus.
- Celebrate Progress: Track your achievements, be it increased weight, improved form, or pain-free movement. Celebrate small victories, stay motivated, and enjoy the journey of building a strong and empowered core.

Remember:

Recovery and maintenance are integral parts of your Windmill journey, not afterthoughts. By prioritizing these practices, you'll cultivate a sustainable training approach, optimize your results, and prevent setbacks. Most importantly, have fun and enjoy the process of building a core that's not just strong, but also resilient and ready for any challenge!

This chapter concludes your comprehensive guide to the Windmill. Remember, consistency, dedication, and the right approach are key to unlocking its transformative power. Embrace the journey, stay true to your goals, and celebrate your success!

Additional Tips:

- Consider incorporating mindfulness practices like meditation or deep breathing to manage stress and promote overall well-being, which can positively impact your Windmill training.
- Explore healthy recipes and meal plans specifically designed for athletes to ensure you're fueling your body optimally for both performance and recovery.
- Join online communities or fitness groups focused on core training or the Windmill exercise specifically. Find motivation, share experiences, and learn from others who are on similar journeys.

Chapter 11

Synergistic Exercises: Complementing the Windmill with Other Core Workouts

The Windmill reigns supreme for sculpting a strong and stable core, but true core mastery demands a well-rounded approach. This chapter delves into synergistic exercises that perfectly complement the Windmill, targeting different core muscles and movement patterns, ensuring a holistic and balanced core training program.

Beyond the Windmill:

While the Windmill offers potent core engagement, incorporating other exercises broadens your training spectrum, preventing plateaus, addressing specific weaknesses, and maximizing core development. Here are some synergistic exercises to consider:

Anti-Rotational Exercises:

- Pallof press: Anchor a resistance band at chest height, stand sideways, and press the band away from your body, resisting rotation. Works on core stability and anti-rotation strength.
- Bird-dog: Start on all fours, extend one arm and opposite leg simultaneously, maintaining a flat back and engaged core. Strengthens core, improves stability, and challenges coordination.

Core Endurance and Stability:

- Plank variations: From high planks to side planks and anti-planks, these variations challenge core endurance and stability in diverse ways.
- Hollow body hold: Lie on your back with lower back pressed to the ground, lift legs and shoulders slightly off the ground, and maintain a "scooped" spine position. Builds core strength and endurance.

Rotational Core Work:

- Russian twists: Sit on the ground with knees bent and feet flat, lean back slightly, and twist your torso from side to side while holding a weight. Targets obliques and rotational core strength.
- Medicine ball slams: Stand tall, hold a medicine ball overhead, and slam it forcefully down to the ground in front of you, engaging your core in the movement. Develops power and rotational core strength.

Remember:

- Choose exercises that complement your Windmill workouts and target areas you want to strengthen or improve.
- Prioritize proper form over heavier weights. Focus on controlled movements and feeling the targeted muscles engage.
- Gradually increase the difficulty or add variations as you progress.
- Listen to your body and take rest days when needed.

Sample Workout:

Warm-up: 5-10 minutes of light cardio and dynamic stretches

Circuit 1 (3 sets of 10-12 repetitions each):

- Windmill (choose weight for moderate challenge)
- Pallof press (each side)
- Bird-dog (each side)

Circuit 2 (3 sets of 30-60 seconds hold each):

- Plank
- Side plank (each side)
- Hollow body hold

Circuit 3 (3 sets of 15-20 repetitions each):

- Russian twists
- Medicine ball slams

Cool-down: 5-10 minutes of static stretches and foam rolling

Remember: This is just a sample. Adapt the exercises, sets, reps, and weights to your fitness level and goals.

Embrace the Synergy:

By incorporating these synergistic exercises alongside your Windmill practice, you unlock a world of core training possibilities. Each exercise contributes to a well-rounded core foundation, building strength, stability, endurance, and power, preparing you for any physical challenge life throws your way. Remember, consistency is key! So, stay motivated, explore different exercises, and enjoy the journey towards a sculpted and empowered core!

Chapter 12

Functional Core Training: Integrating Windmills into Daily Activities and Sports

The true power of the Windmill lies beyond aesthetics and gym sessions. Its core-strengthening magic can translate into your everyday life and athletic endeavors, enhancing performance, preventing injuries, and improving overall movement quality. This chapter explores how to integrate the Windmills into your daily activities and sports routines, unlocking a world of functional core training.

Beyond the Gym:

The Windmill trains your core for real-world movement, not just isolated exercises. By incorporating Windmill principles into your daily life, you can reap the benefits throughout your day:

- Picking up objects: Instead of bending at your back, hinge at your hips and engage your core, mimicking the Windmill movement, to protect your spine.
- Gardening: Utilize the Windmill hinge and core engagement when lifting, weeding, or planting, reducing strain on your lower back.
- Carrying groceries: Distribute weight evenly, engage your core, and maintain a tall posture like in the Windmill to avoid slouching and back pain.
- Playing with kids: Get down on the ground with proper Windmill form (hips back, core engaged) to interact with your children, building core strength and having fun simultaneously.

Sports Synergy:

Windmill training translates beautifully into various sports, improving performance and reducing injury risk:

- Golf: The hinged posture and core engagement in the Windmill resemble the golf swing, promoting power and stability.
- Tennis: The rotational core strength developed with Windmills translates to powerful serves and improved agility on the court.
- Running: A strong core from Windmills improves running posture, reduces fatigue, and enhances overall running efficiency.
- Martial arts: The core stability and power gained from Windmills benefit throws, strikes, and overall balance in martial arts disciplines.

Integration Strategies:

- Warm-up with Windmills: Perform a few modified Windmills with light weight or bodyweight before your sports practice or game to activate your core and prepare for movement.
- Cool-down with Windmills: Include Windmill variations or holds in your

cool-down routine to improve core recovery and flexibility.

- Sport-Specific Adaptations: Consult a coach or trainer to explore how you can adapt Windmill movements specifically for your sport, targeting relevant muscle groups and movement patterns.

Remember:

- Start slow and gradually integrate Windmills into your daily activities and sports routines.
- Listen to your body and adjust the intensity or frequency as needed.
- Don't neglect proper form and core engagement, even outside the gym.
- Enjoy the process! Experiencing the benefits of a strong core in your daily life and athletic pursuits will keep you motivated and inspired.

Embrace the Transformation:

The Windmill is more than just an exercise; it's a gateway to functional core training that empowers you in everyday life and enhances your athletic potential. By integrating Windmill principles into your daily activities and sports, you unlock a world of movement efficiency, injury prevention, and a stronger, more confident you. So, step outside the gym, embrace the functional power of the Windmill, and move with strength, stability, and newfound freedom!

Chapter 13

Advanced Windmill Variations: Pushing Your Limits Safely and Effectively

Conquered the basic Windmill and its synergistic exercises? Ready to delve deeper and challenge your core to new heights? This chapter unveils advanced Windmill variations, designed to push your limits while prioritizing safety and technique. Remember, progression is key, so approach these variations with caution and a focus on proper form.

Advanced Doesn't Mean Reckless:

Before diving in, remember:

- Master the basics first: Ensure you have a solid foundation in the fundamental Windmill before attempting advanced variations.

- Focus on form, not weight: Prioritize perfect form over heavier weights. Incorrect technique can lead to injury, even with lighter weights.
- Listen to your body: Don't push through pain. If you experience discomfort, stop the exercise and consult a healthcare professional.
- Warm-up thoroughly: Prepare your body for the increased challenge with a dynamic warm-up and light Windmill drills.

Variations to Ignite Your Core:

- Single-leg Windmill: Increase core stability and balance by performing the Windmill while balancing on one leg.
- Offset Windmill: Hold the kettlebell offset from your body, adding an anti-rotational challenge to your core.
- Traveling Windmill: Take a small step to the side as you perform the Windmill,

incorporating a dynamic element and challenging your coordination.

- Windmill with rotation: As you reach the bottom of the Windmill, rotate your torso 90 degrees before returning to the starting position.
- Double kettlebell Windmill: Hold a kettlebell in each hand for an extra core and grip strength challenge (advanced!).

Progressive Overload Strategies:

- Increase weight: Gradually increase the weight of the kettlebell as you get stronger.
- Increase reps/sets: Once you can comfortably perform a variation, increase the number of repetitions or sets.
- Decrease rest time: Shorten your rest periods between sets to increase the intensity of your workout.
- Combine variations: Create challenging combinations of different variations to keep your workouts fresh and challenging.

Safety First:

- Use a spotter: When attempting new variations, especially with heavier weights, consider having a spotter to assist you.
- Land softly: Pay attention to your landing on the descent of the Windmill. Land with soft knees and engaged core to avoid impact on your joints.
- Don't force it: If a variation feels uncomfortable or painful, stop immediately and try a different one.

Remember:

Advanced Windmill variations are not for everyone. Consult a certified trainer or physical therapist to assess your suitability and ensure proper technique before attempting them.

Beyond the Chapter:

Remember, the Windmill journey is a continuous exploration. As you progress, consider seeking personalized guidance from professionals, exploring advanced mobility and flexibility drills, and incorporating other core training methods for a well-rounded approach.

Embrace the Challenge:

Advanced Windmill variations offer a thrilling opportunity to push your limits and unlock new levels of core strength and stability. Approach them with dedication, prioritize safety and technique, and enjoy the journey of becoming an even stronger and more empowered individual!

This concludes your comprehensive guide to the Windmill. Remember, consistency, dedication, and the right approach are key to unlocking its transformative power. Embrace the journey, stay true to your goals, and celebrate your success!

Chapter 14

Staying Motivated: Tips and Strategies for Long-Term Adherence

Conquering the Windmill and building a strong core is impressive, but the true test lies in sustained progress. This chapter equips you with essential tips and strategies to stay motivated, overcome plateaus, and make your Windmill practice a lifelong commitment to a healthy and empowered you.

Fueling Your Motivation:

- Set SMART goals: Establish Specific, Measurable, Achievable, Relevant, and Time-bound goals. Celebrate small wins and adjust goals as needed to maintain momentum.

- Find your "why": Revisit your reasons for starting the Windmill journey. Is it improved health, better athletic performance, or simply feeling stronger? Reconnect with your purpose to reignite your fire.
- Make it fun: Explore different Windmill variations, incorporate music you enjoy, or train with a friend to keep your workouts engaging and enjoyable.
- Track your progress: Keep a log of your workouts, reps, weights, and achievements. Seeing your progress is a powerful motivator.
- Reward yourself: Celebrate milestones and personal bests with non-food rewards like a new workout outfit or a relaxing activity.

Combating Plateaus:

- Switch things up: Introduce new Windmill variations, change the workout environment, or try different training methods to avoid monotony.

- Challenge yourself: Gradually increase weight, reps, or sets to keep your body adapting and progressing.
- Seek inspiration: Read fitness articles, watch motivational videos, or follow inspiring fitness accounts to reignite your passion.
- Join a community: Connect with other Windmill enthusiasts online or in person for support, accountability, and shared experiences.
- Take a break: Sometimes, stepping away for a short period can help you return with renewed motivation and focus.

Overcoming Obstacles:

- Listen to your body: Rest when needed, and don't push through pain. Prioritize injury prevention for long-term success.
- Address setbacks: View setbacks as temporary bumps in the road. Learn from

them, adjust your approach, and keep moving forward.

- Embrace challenges: See challenges as opportunities for growth and improvement. Don't get discouraged by temporary difficulties.
- Celebrate non-scale victories: Focus on progress beyond the scale, like increased strength, endurance, or improved form.
- Seek professional help: If you struggle with motivation or face challenges, consider consulting a personal trainer or therapist for guidance and support.

Remember:

Building a strong core and maintaining a consistent Windmill practice is a journey, not a destination. There will be ups and downs, but with the right strategies and unwavering determination, you can stay motivated and achieve your long-term goals.

Embrace the Journey:

Remember, the Windmill is more than just an exercise; it's a commitment to a healthier, stronger, and more empowered you. Embrace the journey, find joy in the process, and celebrate every step forward. With dedication and these valuable tools, you'll cultivate a sustainable Windmill practice that empowers you for life!

This concludes your comprehensive guide to the Windmill. Remember, consistency, dedication, and the right approach are key to unlocking its transformative power. Embrace the journey, stay true to your goals, and celebrate your success!

Chapter 15

Conclusion: Building a Strong, Stable, and Pain-Free Core with Kettlebell Windmills

You've reached the final chapter of your Windmill journey! This comprehensive guide has equipped you with the knowledge, strategies, and inspiration to unlock the transformative power of this exercise and build a strong, stable, and pain-free core.

Key Takeaways:

- The Windmill is a powerful exercise that engages multiple core muscles, promoting stability, strength, and improved movement.
- Proper form and technique are crucial for maximizing benefits and preventing injury.
- Mastering the basic Windmill is essential before exploring advanced variations.

- A well-rounded core training program incorporates other exercises alongside Windmills for holistic development.
- Integrating Windmill principles into daily activities and sports enhances functional core strength and injury prevention.
- Staying motivated and overcoming plateaus requires setting goals, finding joy in the process, and seeking support when needed.

The Windmill Beyond this Guide:

Remember, this guide is just the beginning. As you progress on your Windmill journey, consider:

- Seeking personalized guidance: Consult a certified trainer or physical therapist to tailor your workouts and ensure proper form, especially for advanced variations.
- Exploring advanced mobility and flexibility drills: Enhance your movement

potential and optimize Windmill performance.

- Incorporating other core training methods: Pilates, yoga, or bodyweight exercises can complement your Windmill practice.
- Sharing your journey: Inspire others by sharing your Windmill experience and motivating them to prioritize core health.

The Final Word:

Embrace the Windmill not just as an exercise, but as a philosophy of core strength and mindful movement. Let it empower you to move with confidence, tackle daily challenges with ease, and experience the joy of a strong and healthy body. Remember, consistency is key, celebrate your progress, and most importantly, enjoy the journey towards a core that is not just strong, but truly remarkable.

Congratulations on embarking on this transformative journey! May your Windmill practice continue to empower you and unlock your full potential!

Request for a review

Dear Reader,

I hope you've found "The Pain-Free Core Solution Kettlebell Windmills for a Strong, Stable Midsection, " to be a valuable resource on your journey to mastering this dynamic exercise. Your feedback is immensely important to us, and we would love to hear about your experience with the book.

If you've enjoyed the content, gained insights, or found the information helpful, kindly consider leaving a review. Your thoughts not only contribute to the growth of this guide but also help fellow readers make informed decisions.

Your feedback is highly valued, and we appreciate your time and consideration.

Warm regards,

Helen Talbott